Unexpecte

for Expecting Parents!

Mom and Dad's Edition Pregnancy Journal

MW01268700

@ Journals & Notebooks

@ Journals & Notebooks

Copyright 2016

| Week of | Jan | Feb | Mar | Apr | May | Jun | Jul | Aug | Sep | Oct | Nov | Dec |

Name of the Baby _____

Doctors' Appoinment

Goals

Things to get ready

How do you feel?

Picture here

Memorable experience

Notes

How do you feel?

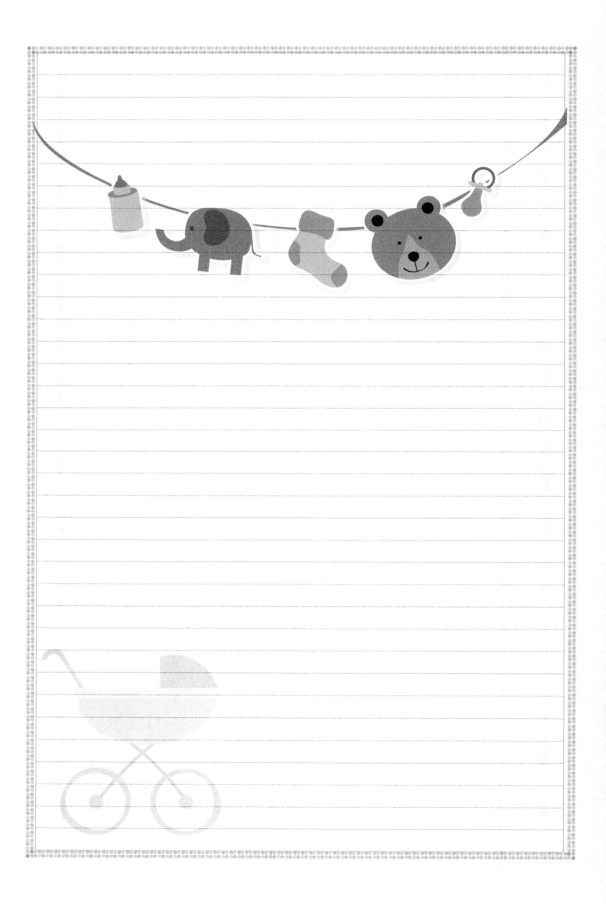

Week of	Jan	Feb	Mar	Apr	May	Jun	Jul	Aug	Sep	Oct	Nov	Dec

Name of the Baby _____

Doctors' Appoinment

Goals

Things to get ready

How do you feel?

Picture here

Memorable experience

Notes

How do you feel?

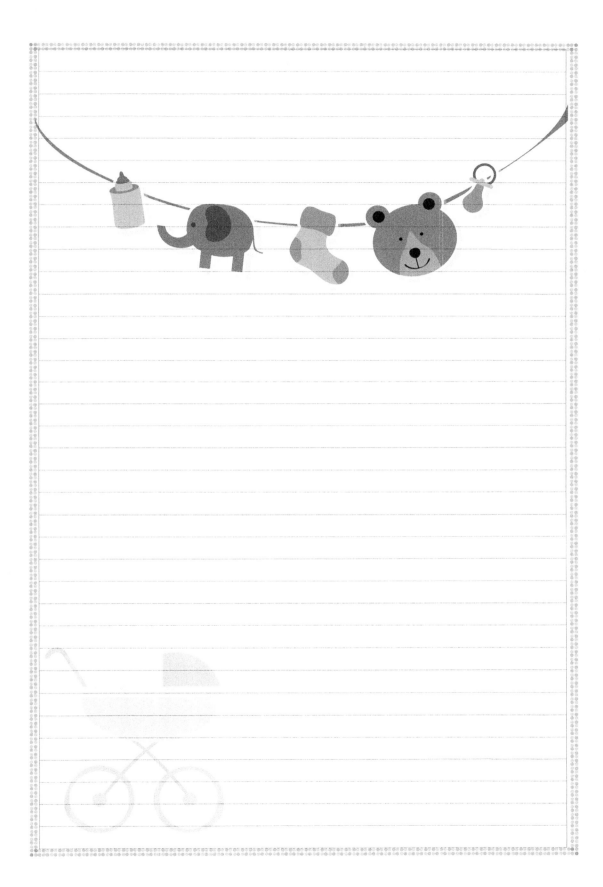

Week of

Jan Feb Mar Apr May Jun Jul Aug Sep Oct Nov Dec

Name of the Baby _____

* * * * * * * * * * * * * * * * * *

Doctors' Appoinment

* * * * * * * * * * * * * * * * * *

Goals

Things to get ready

How do you feel?

Picture here

Memorable experience

Notes

How do you feel?

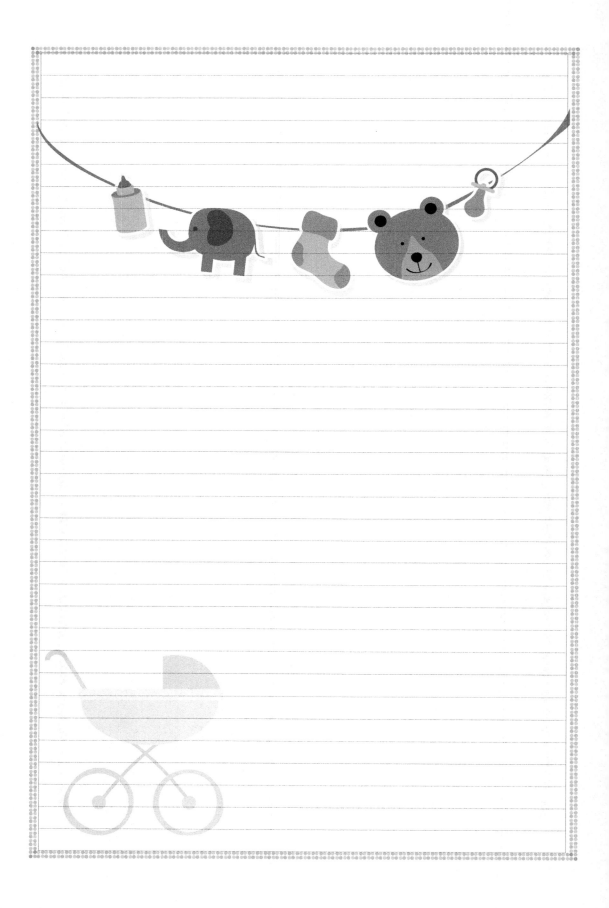

Week of Jan Feb Mar Apr May Jun Jul Aug Sep Oct Nov Dec

Name of the Baby _____

Doctors' Appoinment

Goals

Things to get ready

How do you feel?

Picture here

Memorable experience

Notes

How do you feel?

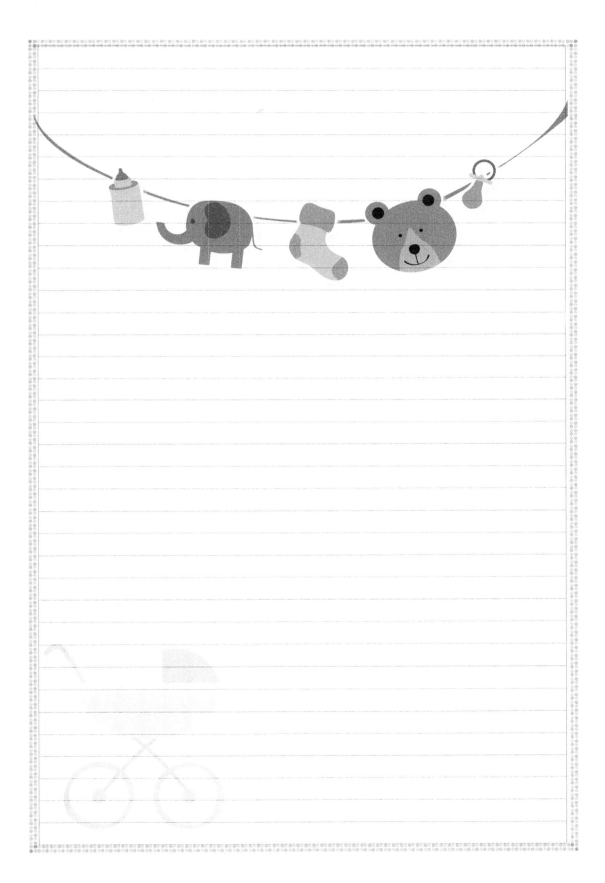

Week of	Jan	Feb	Mar	Apr	May	Jun	Jul	Aug	Sep	Oct	Nov	Dec

Name of the Baby _____

Doctors' Appoinment

Goals

Things to get ready

How do you feel?

Picture here

Memorable experience

Notes

How do you feel?

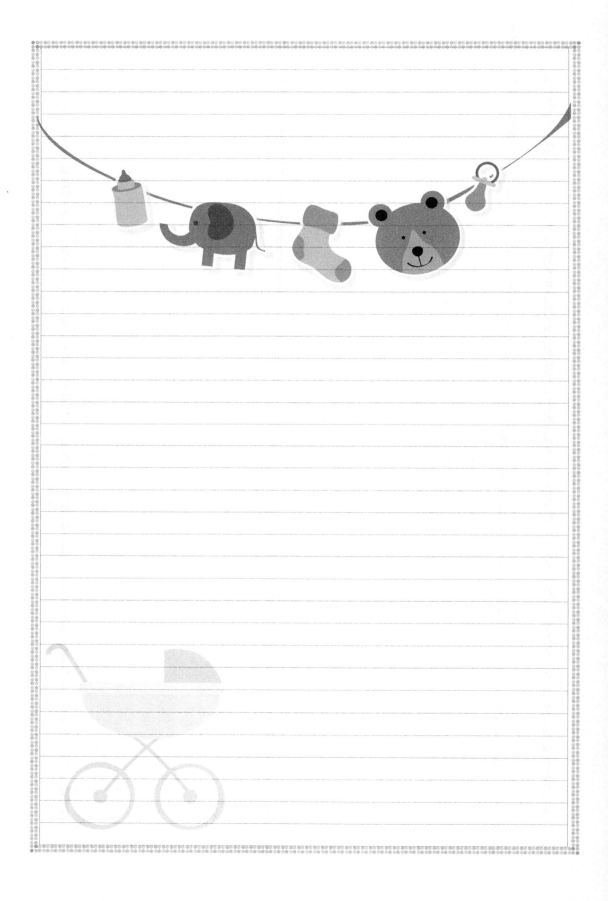

Week of	Jan	Feb	Mar	Apr	May	Jun	Jul	Aug	Sep	Oct	Nov	Dec

Name of the Baby _____

Doctors' Appoinment

Goals

Things to get ready

How do you feel?

Picture here

Memorable experience

Notes

How do you feel?

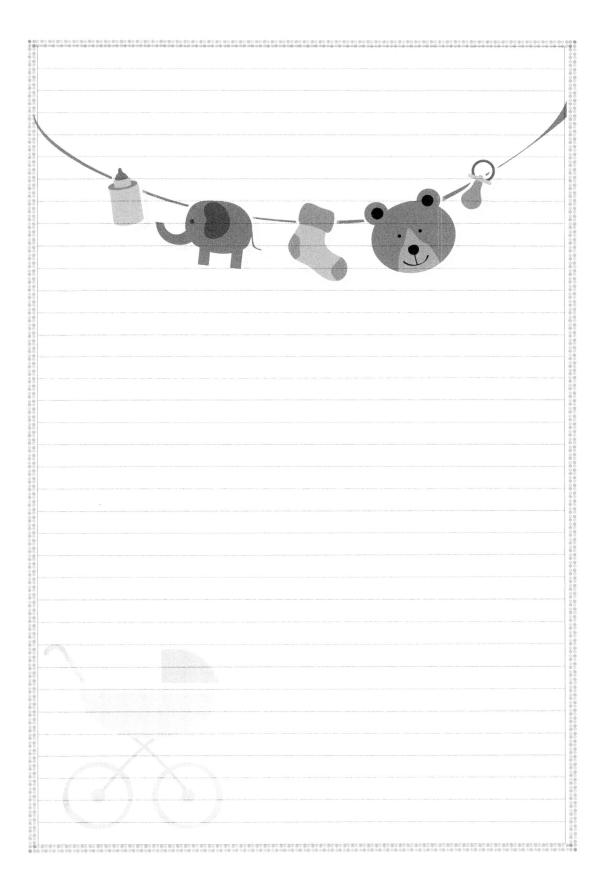

Week of

Name of the Baby _____

Doctors' Appoinment

Goals

Things to get ready

How do you feel?

Picture here

Memorable experience

Notes

How do you feel?

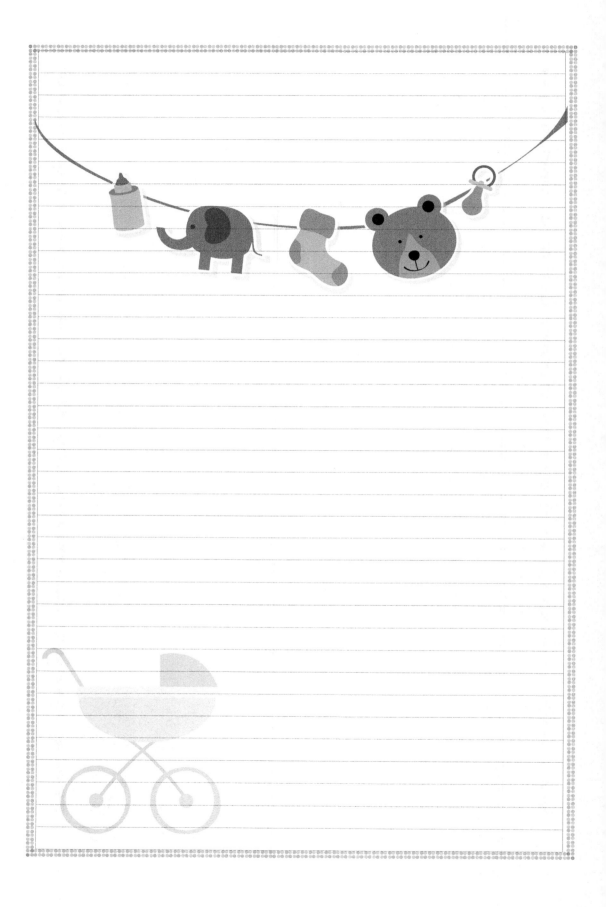

Week of			Jan	Feb	Mar	Apr	May	Jun	Jul	Aug	Sep	Oct	Nov	Dec

Name of the Baby _____

* *

Doctors' Appoinment

* *

Goals

Things to get ready

How do you feel?

Picture here

Memorable experience

Notes

How do you feel?

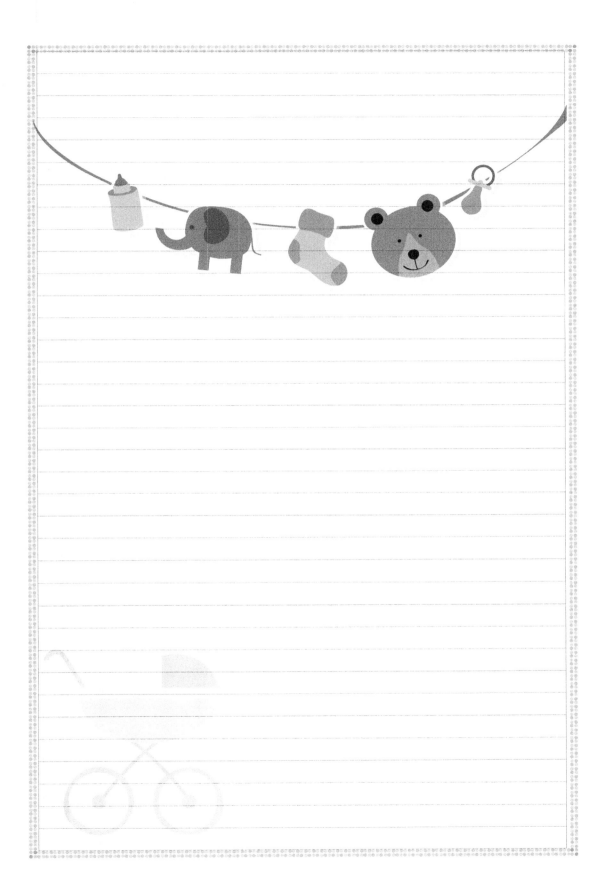

Week of		Jan	Feb	Mar	Apr	May	Jun	Jul	Aug	Sep	Oct	Nov	Dec

Name of the Baby _____

Doctors' Appoinment

Goals

Things to get ready

How do you feel?

Picture here

Memorable experience

Notes

How do you feel?

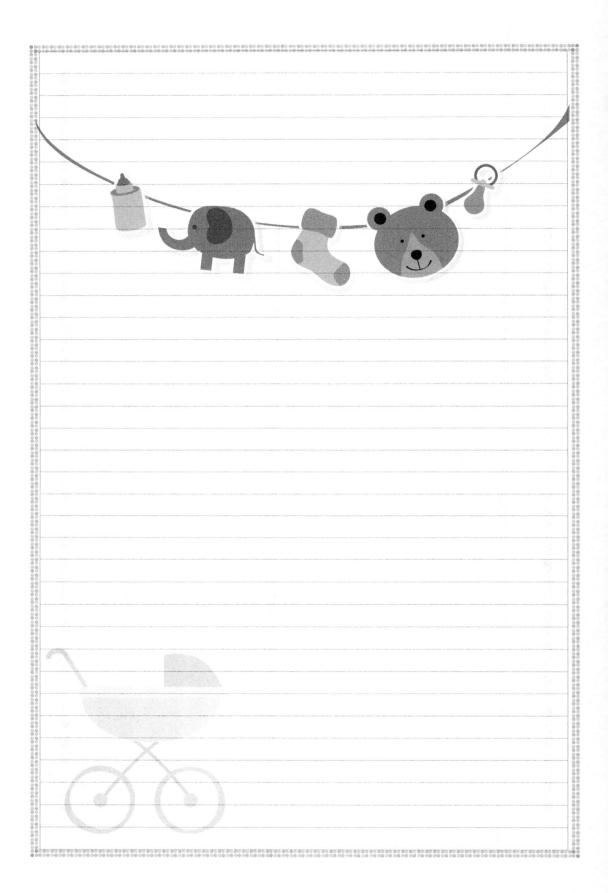

Week of	Jan	Feb	Mar	Apr	May	Jun	Jul	Aug	Sep	Oct	Nov	Dec

Name of the Baby _____

Doctors' Appoinment

Goals

Things to get ready

How do you feel?

Picture here

Memorable experience

Notes

How do you feel?

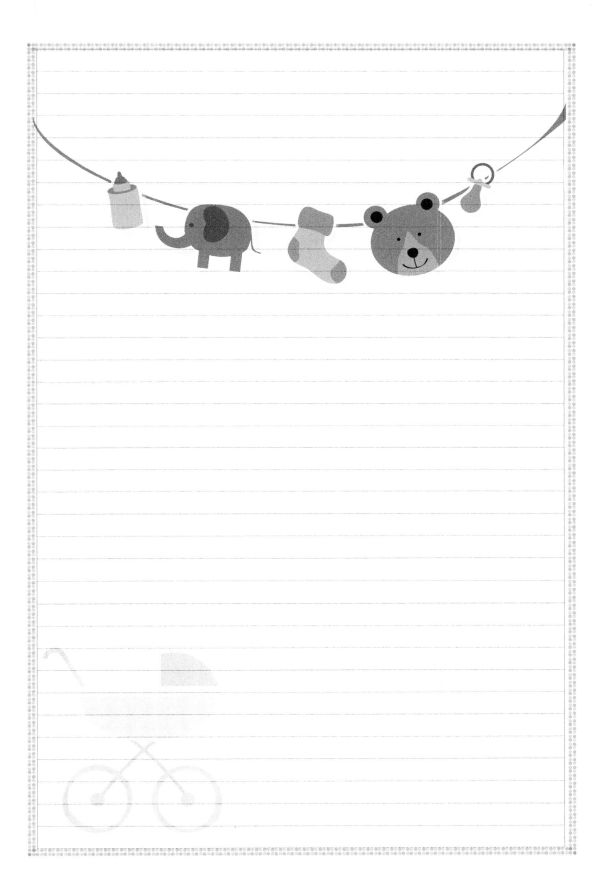

Week of		Jan	Feb	Mar	Apr	May	Jun	Jul	Aug	Sep	Oct	Nov	Dec

Name of the Baby _____

Doctors' Appoinment

Goals

Things to get ready

How do you feel?

Picture here

Memorable experience

Notes

How do you feel?

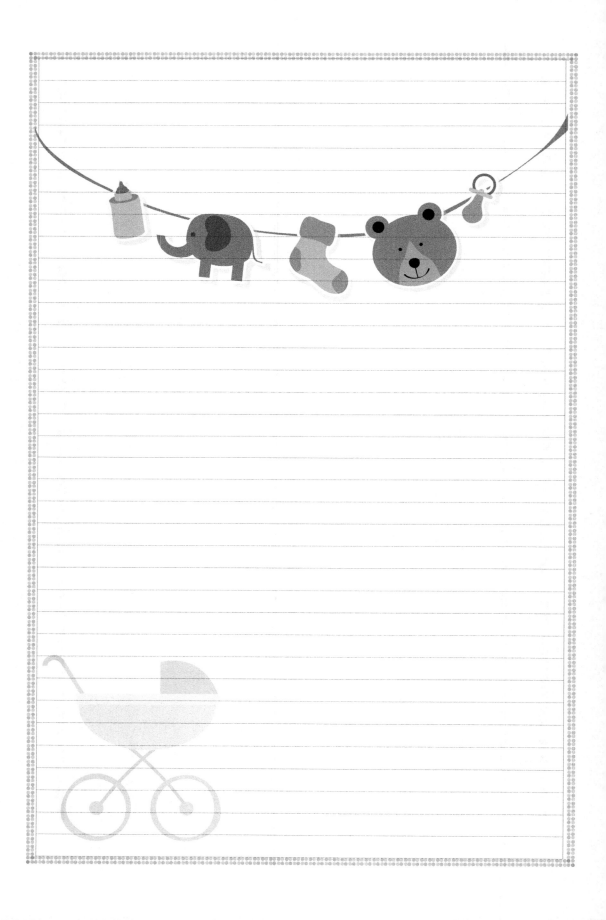

Week of	Jan	Feb	Mar	Apr	May	Jun	Jul	Aug	Sep	Oct	Nov	Dec

Name of the Baby _____

Doctors' Appoinment

Goals

Things to get ready

How do you feel?

Picture here

Memorable experience

Notes

How do you feel?

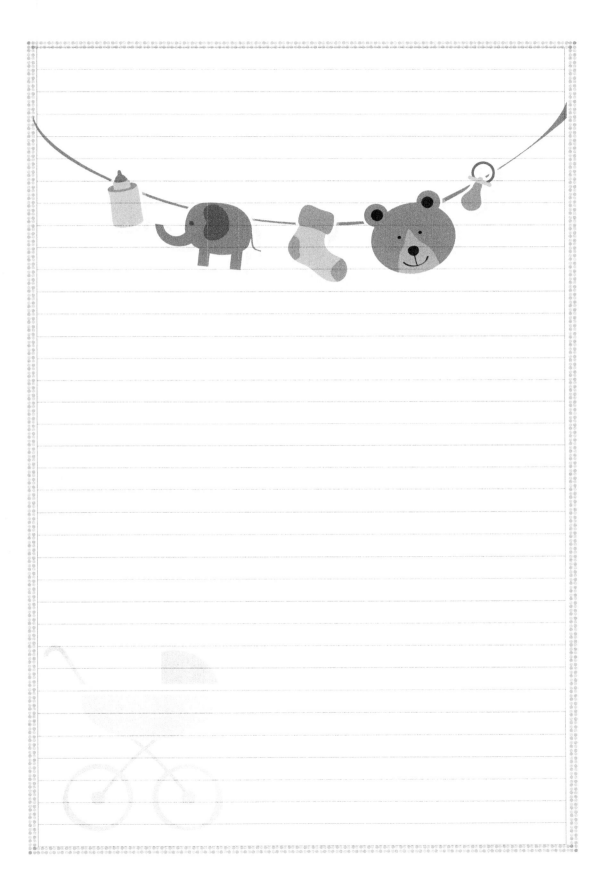

Week of		Jan	Feb	Mar	Apr	May	Jun	Jul	Aug	Sep	Oct	Nov	Dec

Name of the Baby _____

Doctors' Appoinment

Goals

Things to get ready

How do you feel?

Picture here

Memorable experience

Notes

How do you feel?

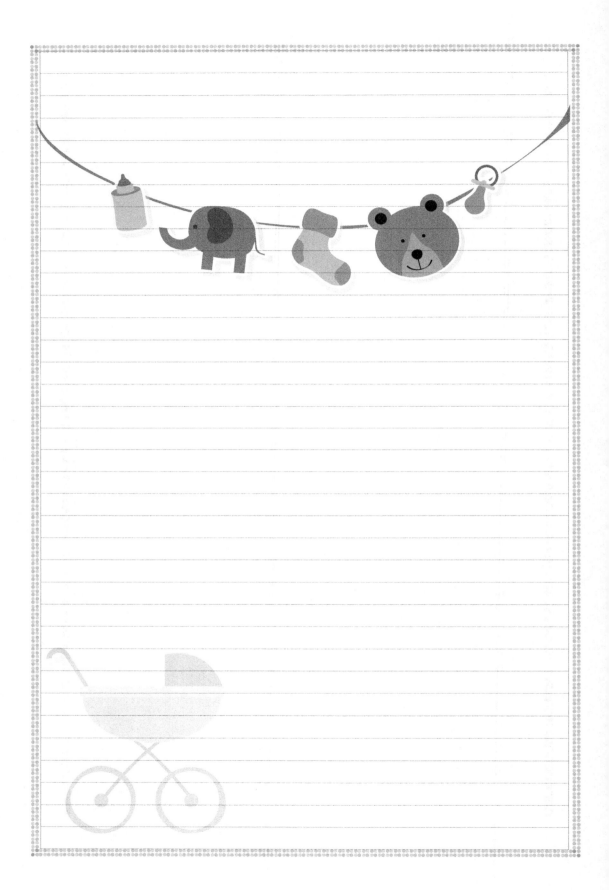

Jan Feb Mar Apr May Jun Jul Aug Sep Oct Nov Dec

Name of the Baby _____

Doctors' Appoinment

Goals

Things to get ready

How do you feel?

Picture here

Memorable experience

Notes

How do you feel?

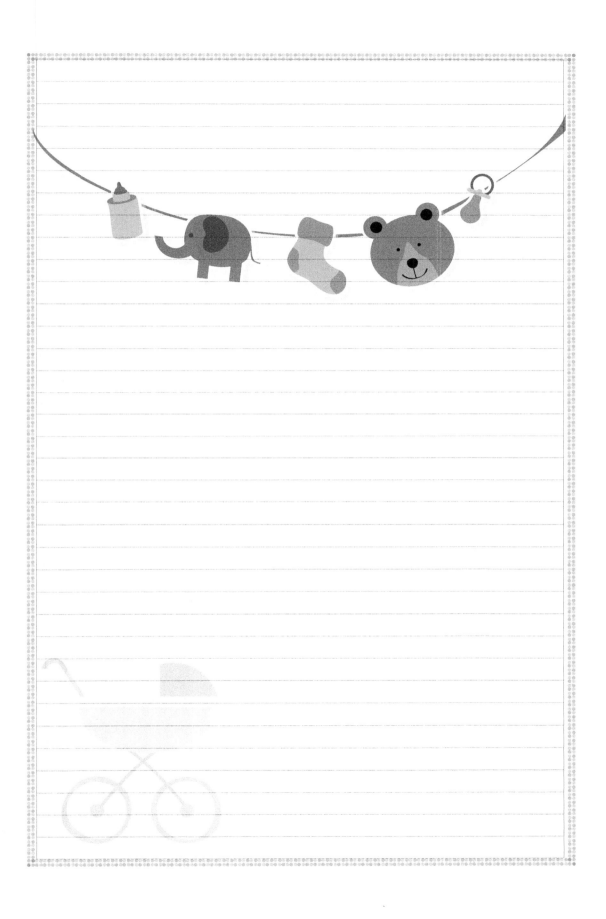

Week of	Jan	Feb	Mar	Apr	May	Jun	Jul	Aug	Sep	Oct	Nov	Dec

Name of the Baby _____

Doctors' Appoinment

Goals

Things to get ready

How do you feel?

Picture here

Memorable experience

Notes

How do you feel?

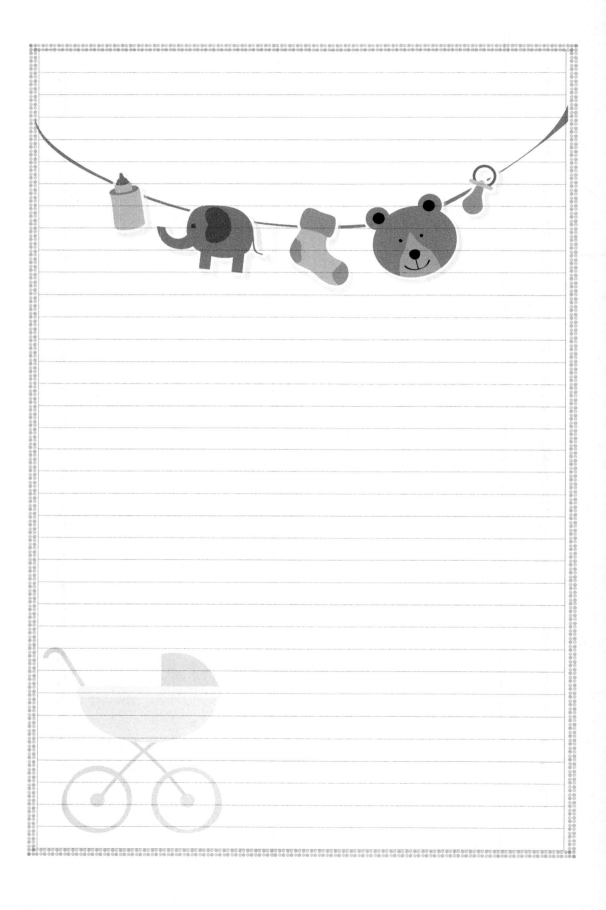

Week of	Jan	Feb	Mar	Apr	May	Jun	Jul	Aug	Sep	Oct	Nov	Dec

Name of the Baby _____

Doctors' Appoinment

Goals

Things to get ready

How do you feel?

Picture here

Memorable experience

Notes

How do you feel?

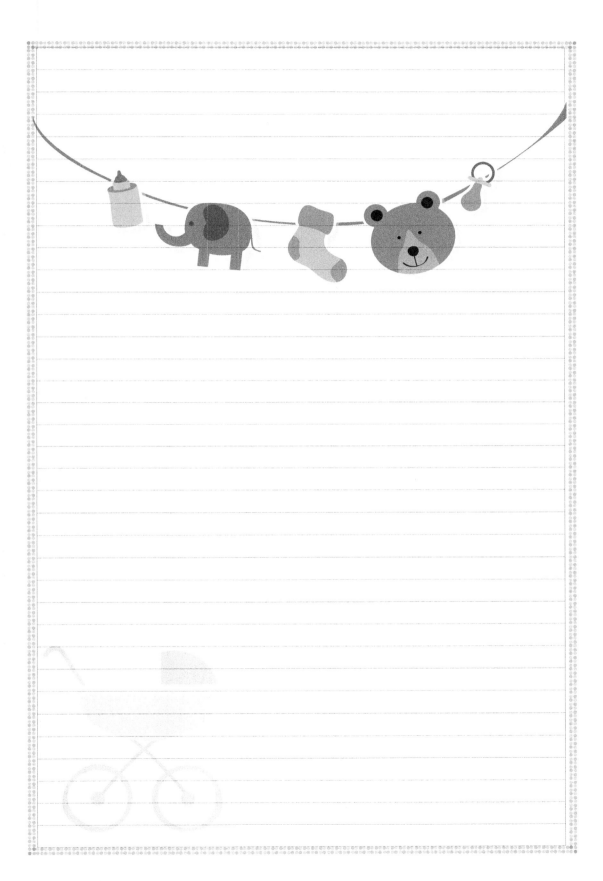

Week of

Jan Feb Mar Apr May Jun Jul Aug Sep Oct Nov Dec

Name of the Baby _____

* *

Doctors' Appoinment

* *

Goals

Things to get ready

How do you feel?

Picture here

Memorable experience

Notes

How do you feel?

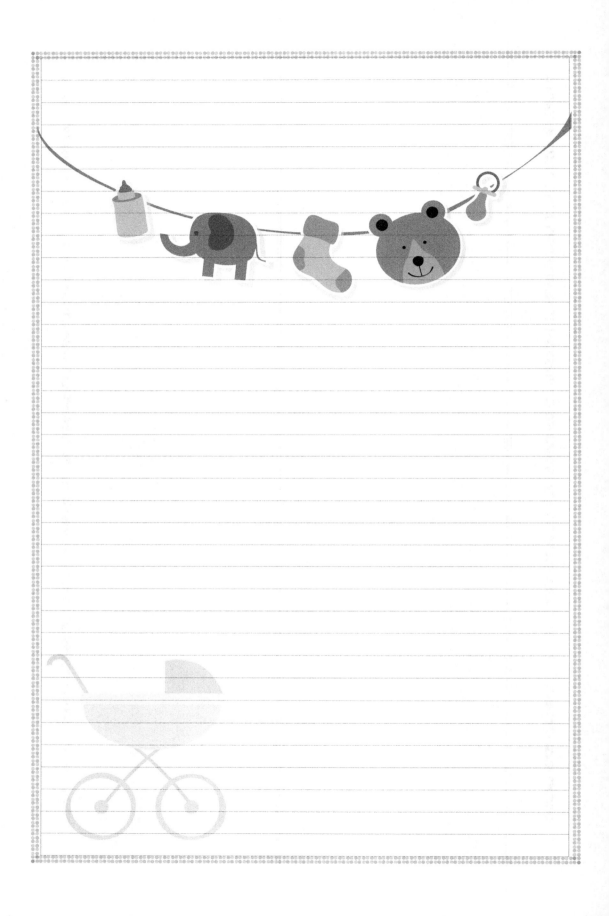

Week of	Jan	Feb	Mar	Apr	May	Jun	Jul	Aug	Sep	Oct	Nov	Dec

Name of the Baby _____

Doctors' Appoinment

Goals

Things to get ready

How do you feel?

Picture here

Memorable experience

Notes

How do you feel?

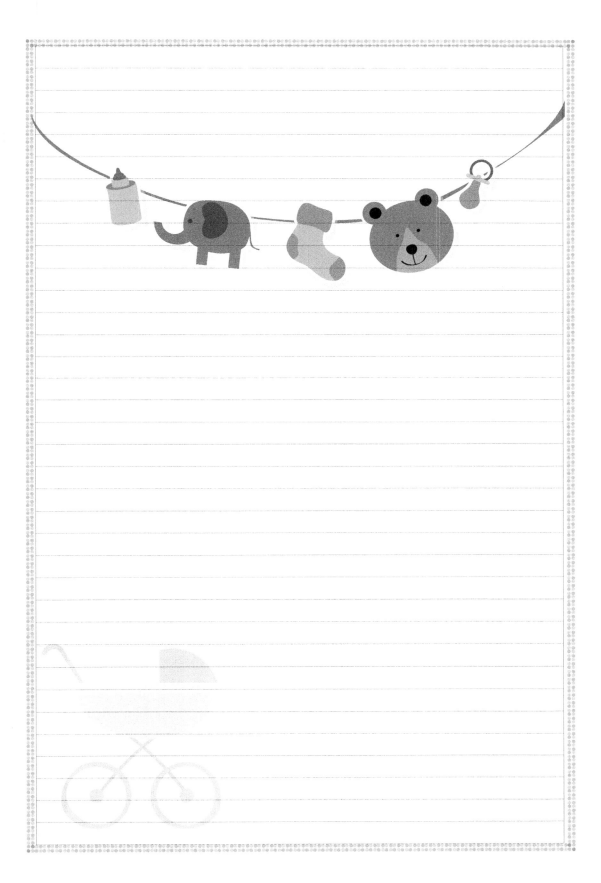

Week of	Jan	Feb	Mar	Apr	May	Jun	Jul	Aug	Sep	Oct	Nov	Dec

Name of the Baby _____

Doctors' Appoinment

Goals

Things to get ready

How do you feel?

Picture here

Memorable experience

Notes

How do you feel?

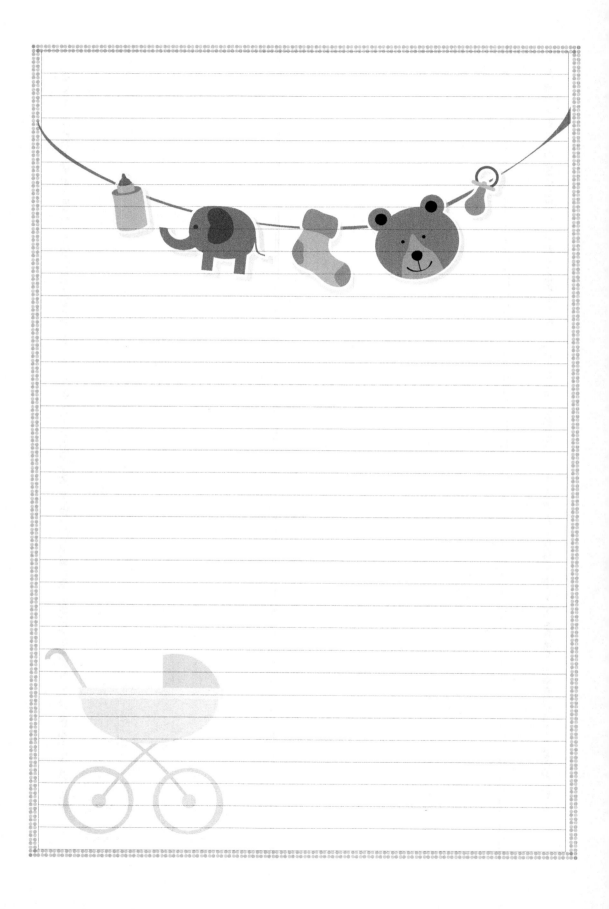

Week of	Jan	Feb	Mar	Apr	May	Jun	Jul	Aug	Sep	Oct	Nov	Dec

Name of the Baby _____

Doctors' Appoinment

Goals

Things to get ready

How do you feel?

Picture here

Memorable experience

Notes

How do you feel?

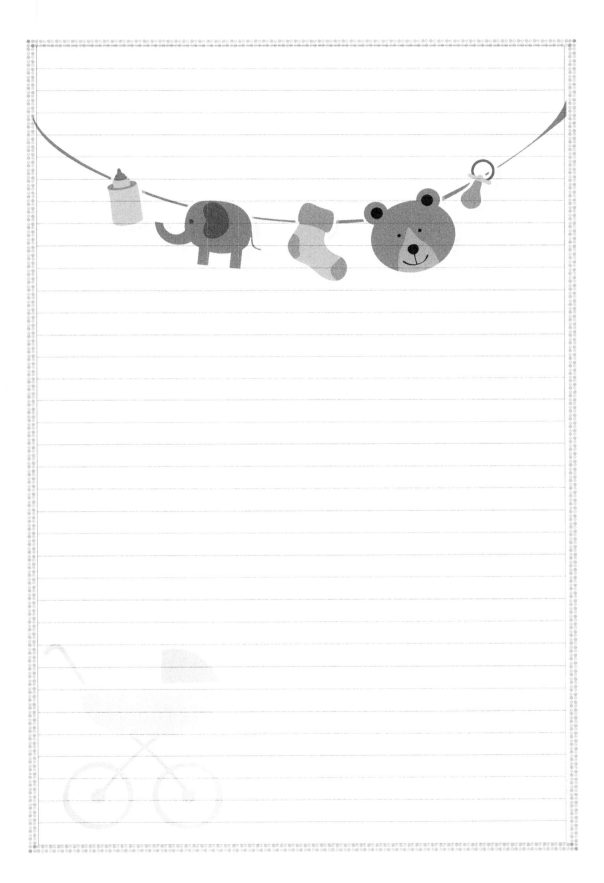

Week of	Jan	Feb	Mar	Apr	May	Jun	Jul	Aug	Sep	Oct	Nov	Dec

Name of the Baby _____

Doctors' Appoinment

Goals

Things to get ready

How do you feel?

Picture here

Memorable experience

Notes

How do you feel?

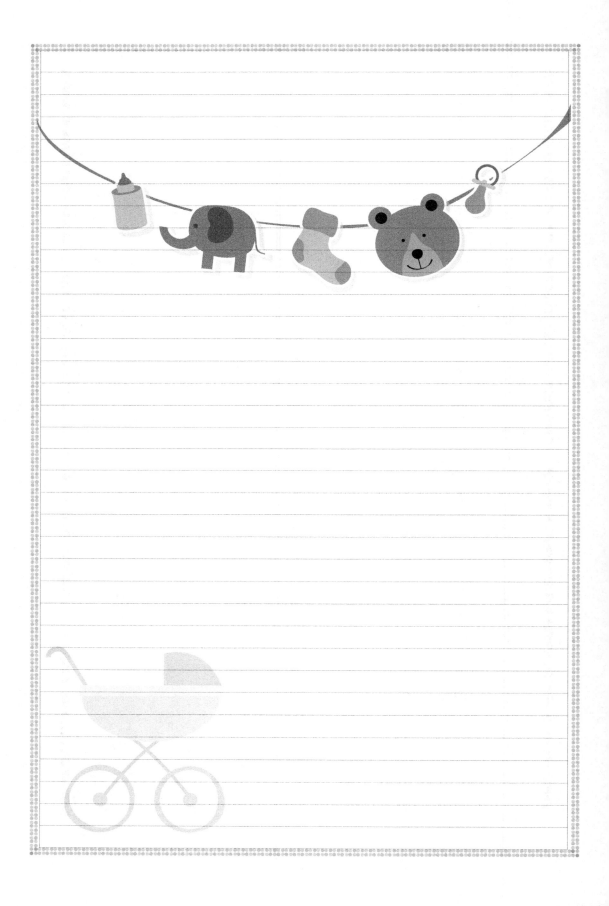

Week of	Jan	Feb	Mar	Apr	May	Jun	Jul	Aug	Sep	Oct	Nov	Dec

Name of the Baby _____

Doctors' Appoinment

Goals

Things to get ready

How do you feel?

Picture here

Memorable experience

Notes

How do you feel?

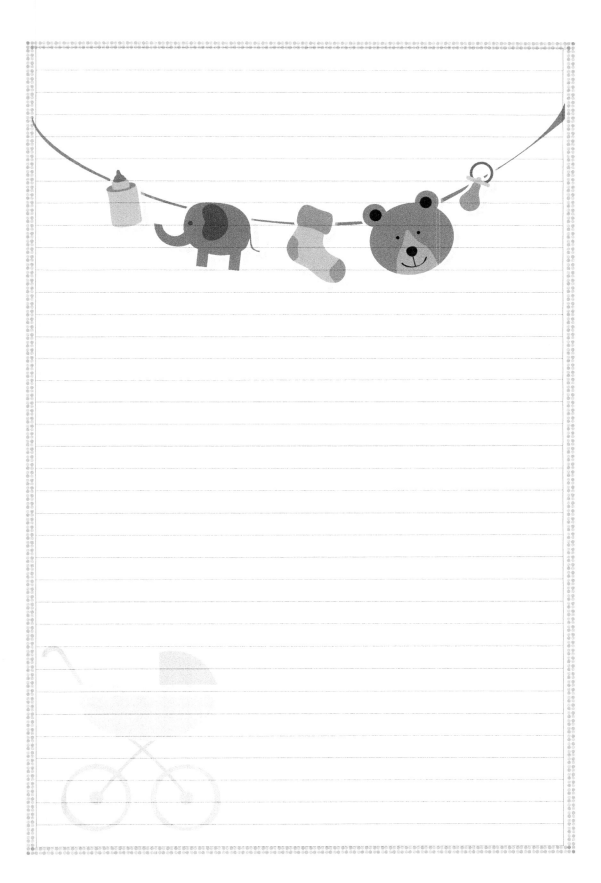

Week of	Jan	Feb	Mar	Apr	May	Jun	Jul	Aug	Sep	Oct	Nov	Dec

Name of the Baby _____

Doctors' Appoinment

Goals

Things to get ready

How do you feel?

Picture here

Memorable experience

Notes

How do you feel?

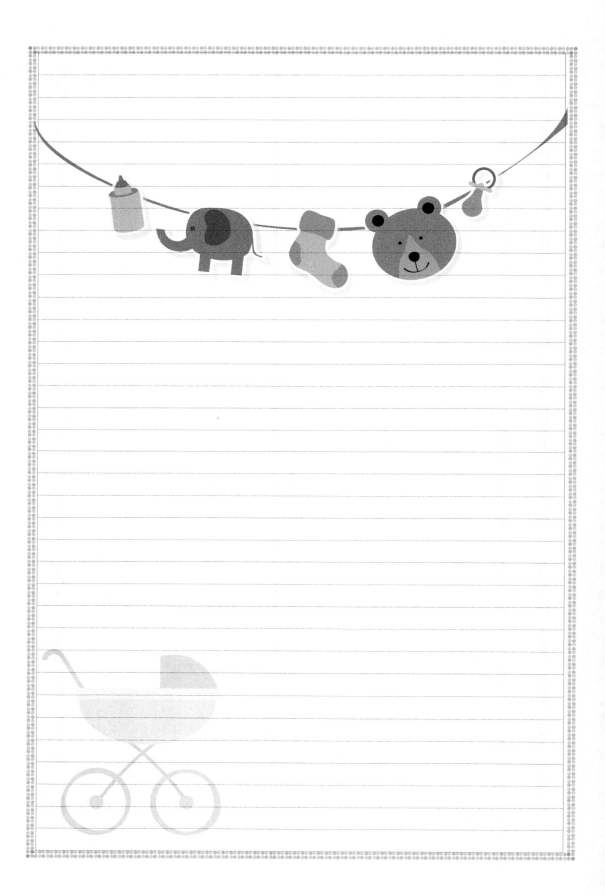

Week of	Jan	Feb	Mar	Apr	May	Jun	Jul	Aug	Sep	Oct	Nov	Dec

Name of the Baby _____

Doctors' Appoinment

Goals

Things to get ready

How do you feel?

Picture here

Memorable experience

Notes

How do you feel?

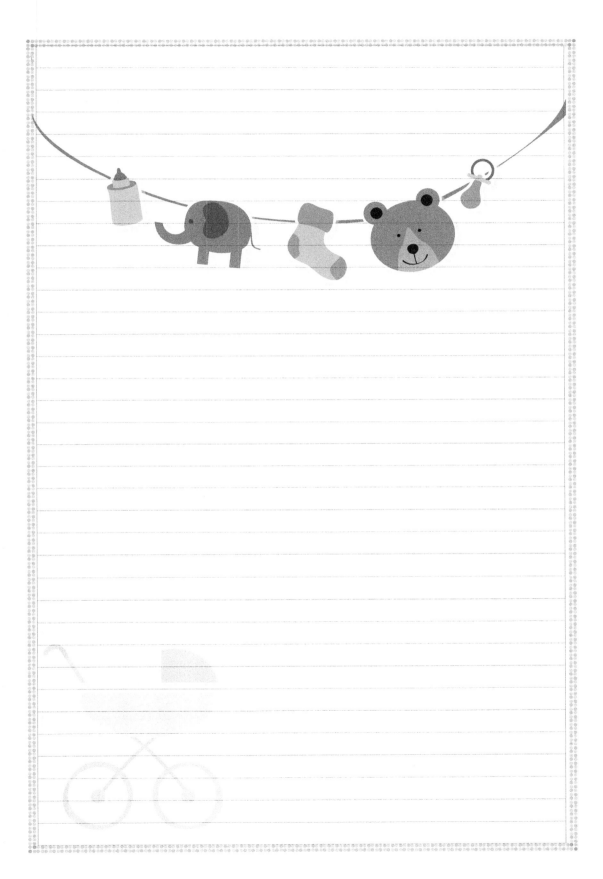

Week of	Jan	Feb	Mar	Apr	May	Jun	Jul	Aug	Sep	Oct	Nov	Dec

Name of the Baby _____

Doctors' Appoinment

Goals

Things to get ready

How do you feel?

Picture here

Memorable experience

Notes

How do you feel?

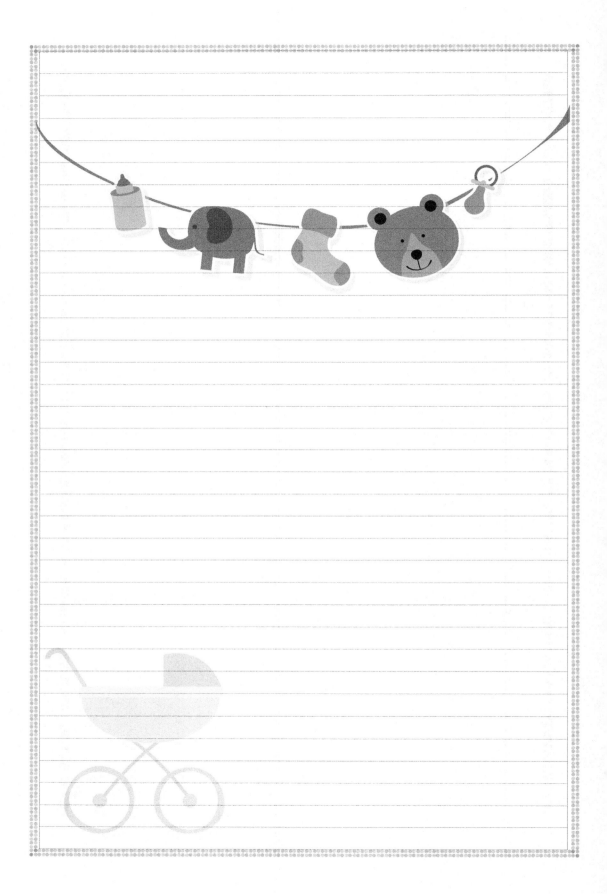

Jan Feb Mar Apr May Jun Jul Aug Sep Oct Nov Dec

Name of the Baby _____

Doctors' Appoinment

Goals

Things to get ready

How do you feel?

Picture here

Memorable experience

Notes

How do you feel?

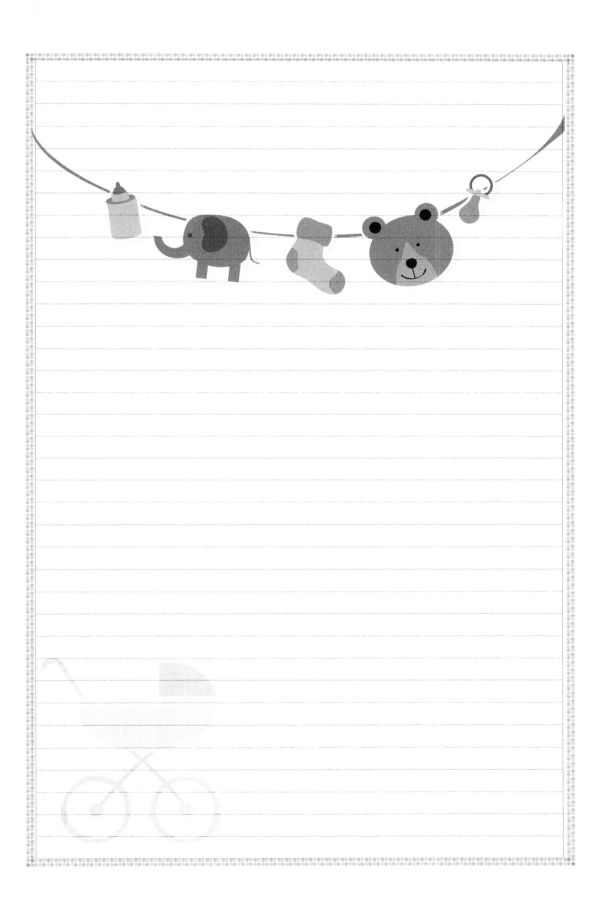

Week of

Name of the Baby _____

Doctors' Appoinment

Goals

Things to get ready

How do you feel?

Picture here

Memorable experience

Notes

How do you feel?

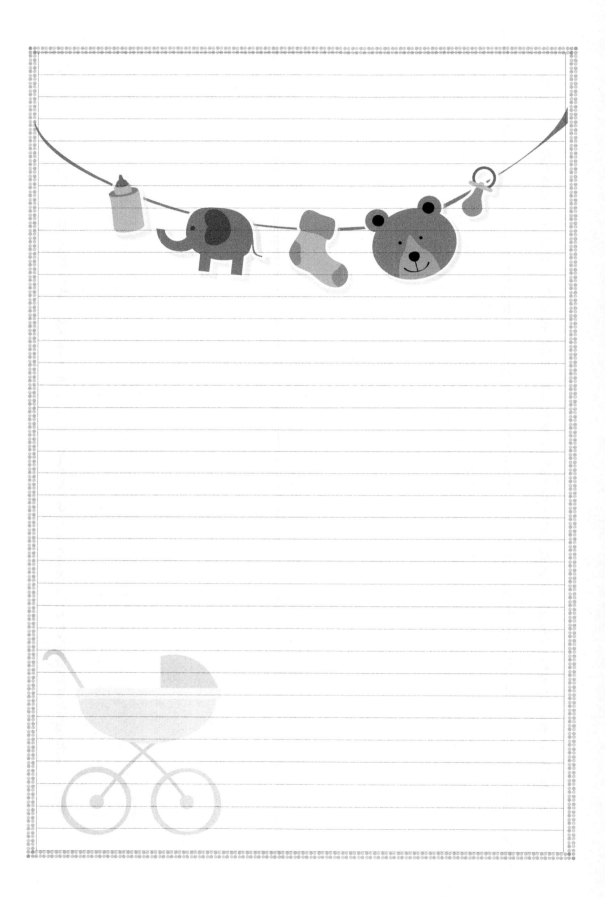

Week of	Jan	Feb	Mar	Apr	May	Jun	Jul	Aug	Sep	Oct	Nov	Dec

Name of the Baby _____

Doctors' Appoinment

Goals

Things to get ready

How do you feel?

Picture here

Memorable experience

Notes

How do you feel?

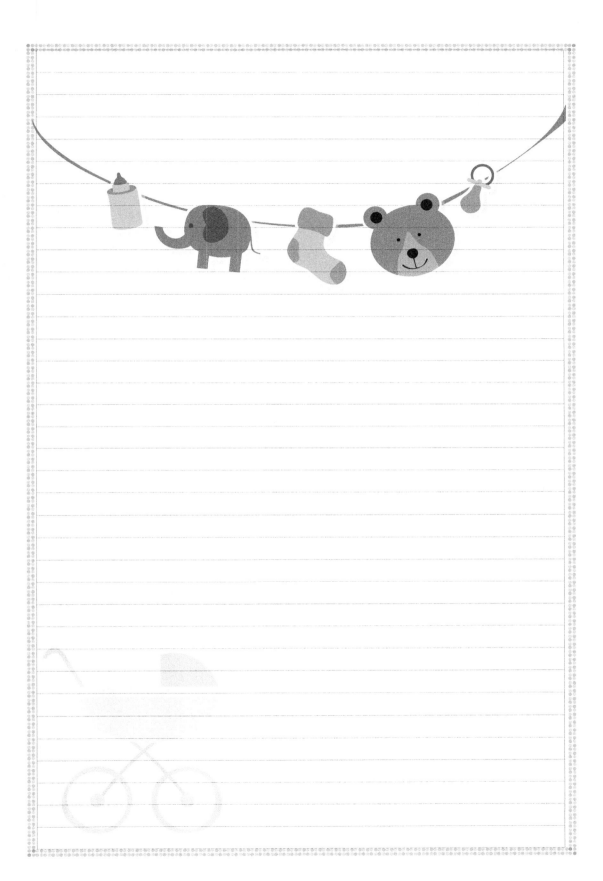

Week of	Jan	Feb	Mar	Apr	May	Jun	Jul	Aug	Sep	Oct	Nov	Dec

Name of the Baby _____

Doctors' Appoinment

Goals

Things to get ready

How do you feel?

Picture here

Memorable experience

Notes

How do you feel?

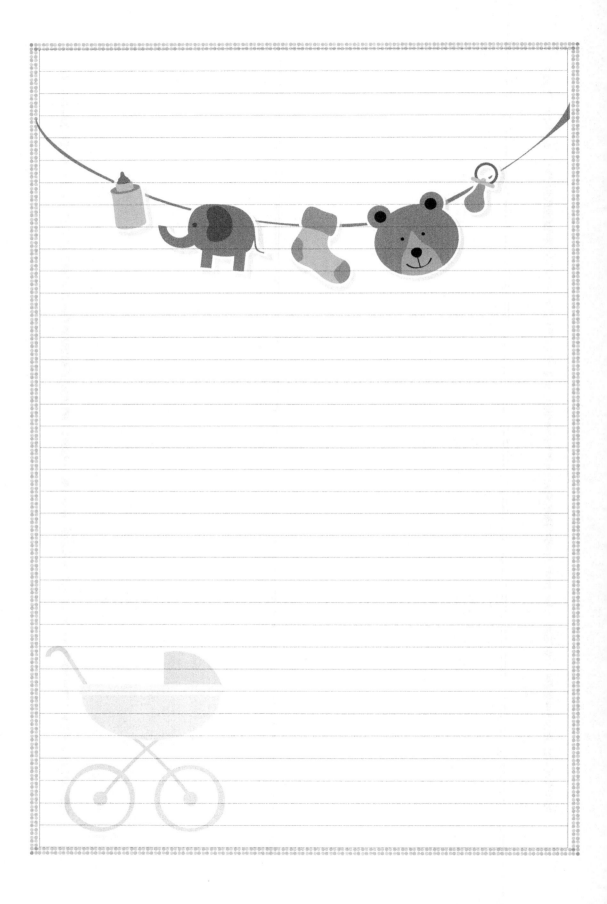

Name of the Baby _____

Doctors' Appoinment

Goals

Things to get ready

How do you feel?

Picture here

Memorable experience

Notes

How do you feel?

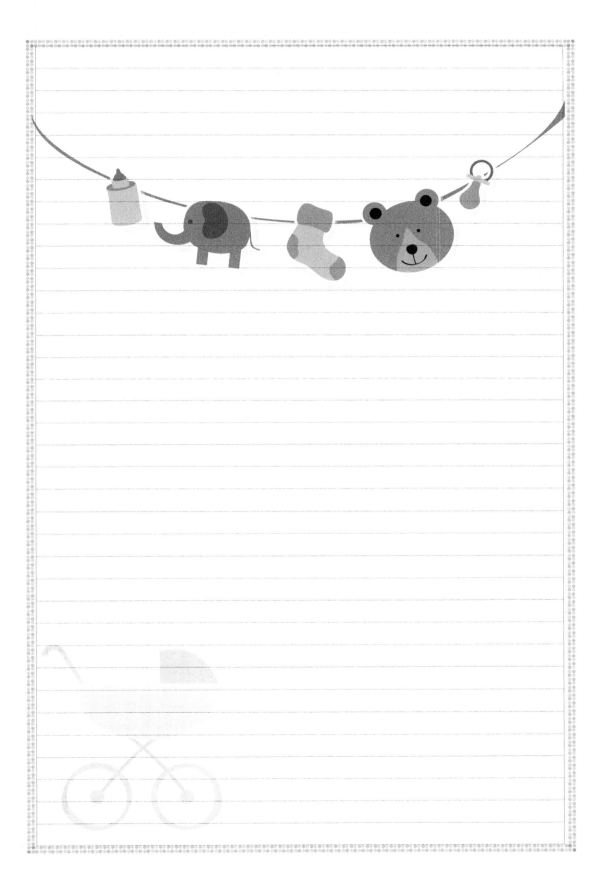

Week of	Jan	Feb	Mar	Apr	May	Jun	Jul	Aug	Sep	Oct	Nov	Dec

Name of the Baby _____

Doctors' Appoinment

Goals

Things to get ready

How do you feel?

Picture here

Memorable experience

Notes

How do you feel?

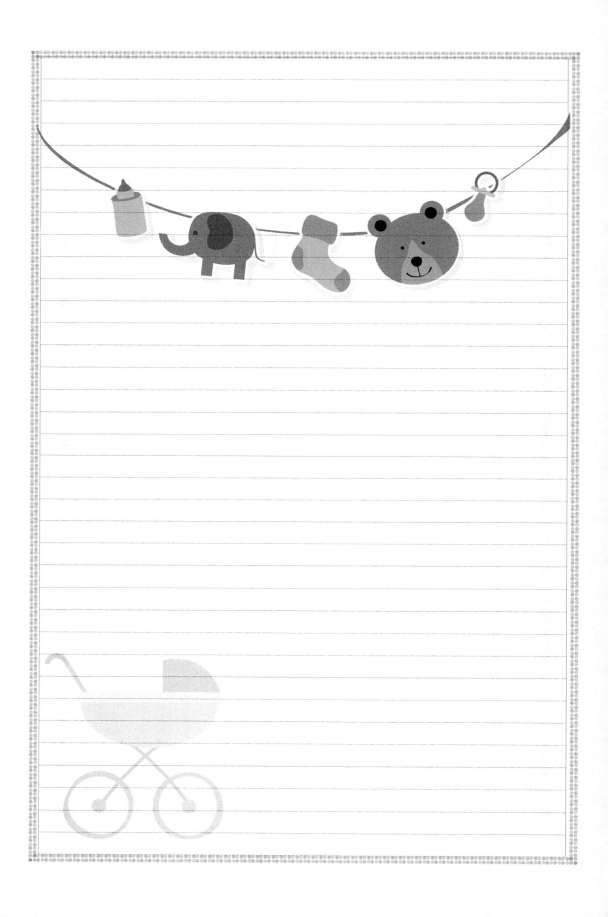

Name of the Baby _____

Doctors' Appoinment

Goals

Things to get ready

How do you feel?

Picture here

Memorable experience

Notes

How do you feel?

| Week of | Jan Feb Mar Apr May Jun Jul Aug Sep Oct Nov Dec |

Name of the Baby _____

Doctors' Appoinment

Goals

Things to get ready

How do you feel?

Picture here

Memorable experience

Notes

How do you feel?

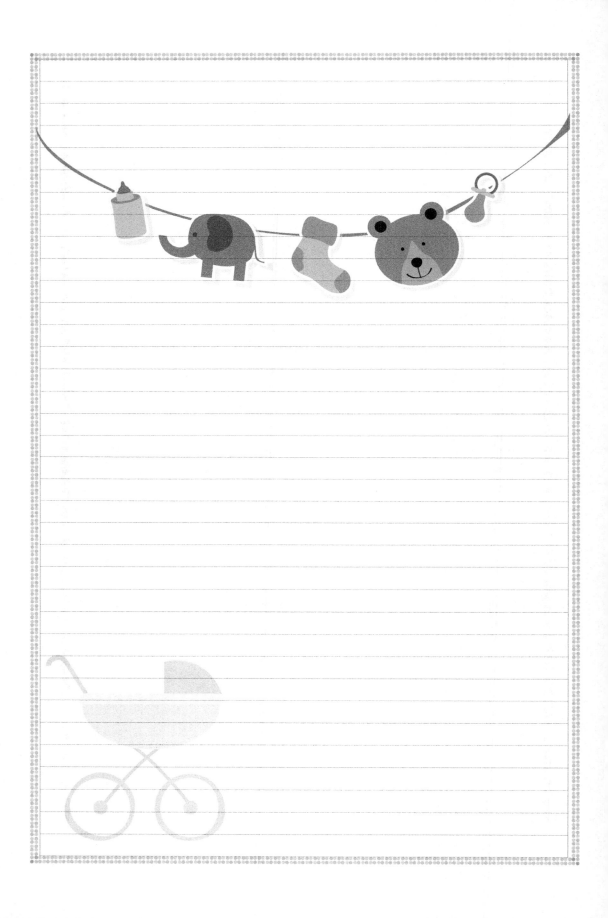

Week of	Jan	Feb	Mar	Apr	May	Jun	Jul	Aug	Sep	Oct	Nov	Dec

Name of the Baby _____

Doctors' Appoinment

Goals

Things to get ready

How do you feel?

Picture here

Memorable experience

Notes

How do you feel?

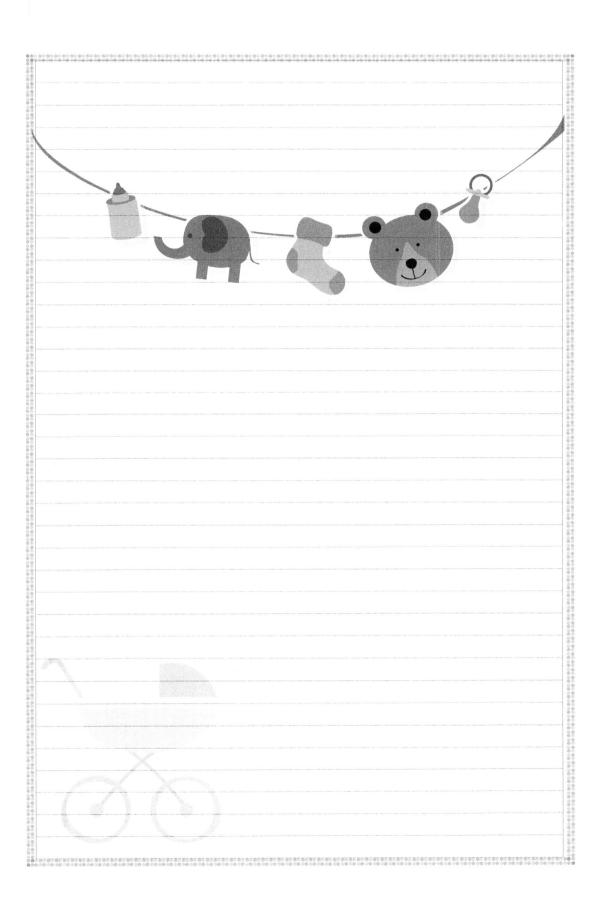

| Week of | Jan | Feb | Mar | Apr | May | Jun | Jul | Aug | Sep | Oct | Nov | Dec |

Name of the Baby _____

* *

Doctors' Appoinment

* *

Goals

Things to get ready

How do you feel?

Picture here

Memorable experience

Notes

How do you feel?

Made in the USA
Las Vegas, NV
14 December 2021

37680816R00059